Workout
Planner

This planner belongs to

30 Day Challenge

Day 1	Day 2	Day 3	Day 4

Day 8	Day 9	Day 10	Day 11

Day 15	Day 16	Day 17	Day 18

Day 22	Day 23	Day 24	Day 25

Day 29	Day 30	Goals

Starts on _____   Ends on _____

Day 5	Day 6	Day 7	Notes

Day 12	Day 13	Day 14	

Day 19	Day 20	Day 21	

Day 26	Day 27	Day 28	

Action plan

- ☐ _____
- ☐ _____
- ☐ _____
- ☐ _____
- ☐ _____

Rewards

30 Day Challenge

Day 1	Day 2	Day 3	Day 4

Day 8	Day 9	Day 10	Day 11

Day 15	Day 16	Day 17	Day 18

Day 22	Day 23	Day 24	Day 25

Day 29	Day 30	Goals

Day 5	Day 6	Day 7	Notes

Day 12	Day 13	Day 14	

Day 19	Day 20	Day 21	

Day 26	Day 27	Day 28	

Action plan

- ☐ _____
- ☐ _____
- ☐ _____
- ☐ _____
- ☐ _____

Rewards

30 Day Challenge

Day 1	Day 2	Day 3	Day 4

Day 8	Day 9	Day 10	Day 11

Day 15	Day 16	Day 17	Day 18

Day 22	Day 23	Day 24	Day 25

Day 29	Day 30	Goals

Starts on _____   Ends on _____

Day 5	Day 6	Day 7	Notes

Day 12	Day 13	Day 14	

Day 19	Day 20	Day 21	

Day 26	Day 27	Day 28	

Action plan

☐ _____

☐ _____

☐ _____

☐ _____

☐ _____

Rewards

Daily Workout

Date _____

Goal

Notes

Water ⬡⬡⬡⬡⬡⬡⬡   Mood 😀 🙂 😊 😒 😰 😖

Meal	Food	Amount	Calories
Breakfast			
Lunch			
Dinner			
Snacks			
		Total	

Workout	Set	Weight	Reps	Distance	Duration	Calories Burned
					Total	

Daily Workout

Date _____

Goal

Notes

Water ⬡ ⬡ ⬡ ⬡ ⬡ ⬡ ⬡ ⬡

Mood 😀 🙂 😊 😐 😣 😵

Meal	Food	Amount	Calories
Breakfast			
Lunch			
Dinner			
Snacks			
		Total	

Workout	Set	Weight	Reps	Distance	Duration	Calories Burned
					Total	

Daily Workout

Date _____

Goal

Notes

Water ◇◇◇◇◇◇◇◇   Mood 😀 🙂 😅 😒 😰 😖

Meal	Food	Amount	Calories
Breakfast			
Lunch			
Dinner			
Snacks			
		Total	

Workout	Set	Weight	Reps	Distance	Duration	Calories Burned
					Total	

Daily Workout

Date _____

Goal	Notes

Water ⬦⬦⬦⬦⬦⬦⬦⬦   Mood 😀 🙂 😊 😌 😰 😵

Meal	Food	Amount	Calories
Breakfast			
Lunch			
Dinner			
Snacks			
		Total	

Workout	Set	Weight	Reps	Distance	Duration	Calories Burned
					Total	

Daily Workout

Date _____

Goal

Notes

Water ⬡ ⬡ ⬡ ⬡ ⬡ ⬡ ⬡   Mood 😀 🙂 😊 😔 😣 😵

Meal	Food	Amount	Calories
Breakfast			
Lunch			
Dinner			
Snacks			
		Total	

Workout	Set	Weight	Reps	Distance	Duration	Calories Burned
					Total	

Daily Workout

Date _____

Goal	Notes

Water ⬦⬦⬦⬦⬦⬦⬦   Mood 😀 🙂 😄 😑 😰 😵

Meal	Food	Amount	Calories
Breakfast			
Lunch			
Dinner			
Snacks			
		Total	

Workout	Set	Weight	Reps	Distance	Duration	Calories Burned
					Total	

Daily Workout

Date _____

Goal

Notes

Water ⬦⬦⬦⬦⬦⬦⬦⬦ Mood 😀 🙂 😊 😑 😖 😵

Meal	Food	Amount	Calories
Breakfast			
Lunch			
Dinner			
Snacks			
		Total	

Workout	Set	Weight	Reps	Distance	Duration	Calories Burned
					Total	

Weekly check in

Week of _____

Goals

Notes

	Mon	Tue	Wed	Thu	Fri	Sat	Sun
Cardio	☐	☐	☐	☐	☐	☐	☐
Arms	☐	☐	☐	☐	☐	☐	☐
Abs and Obliques	☐	☐	☐	☐	☐	☐	☐
Lower body	☐	☐	☐	☐	☐	☐	☐
Rest	☐	☐	☐	☐	☐	☐	☐
Water	☐	☐	☐	☐	☐	☐	☐
Healthy food	☐	☐	☐	☐	☐	☐	☐
	☐	☐	☐	☐	☐	☐	☐
	☐	☐	☐	☐	☐	☐	☐
	☐	☐	☐	☐	☐	☐	☐

	Starting	Ending	Difference	Notes
Weight				
Arms				
Chest				
Waist				
Hips				
Thighs				

Daily Workout

Date _____

Goal

Notes

Water 〇〇〇〇〇〇〇〇   Mood 😀 🙂 😊 😔 😰 😵

Meal	Food	Amount	Calories
Breakfast			
Lunch			
Dinner			
Snacks			
		Total	

Workout	Set	Weight	Reps	Distance	Duration	Calories Burned
					Total	

Daily Workout

Date _____

Goal

Notes

Water ◇◇◇◇◇◇◇◇　　Mood 😀 🙂 😊 😐 😣 😵

Meal	Food	Amount	Calories
Breakfast			
Lunch			
Dinner			
Snacks			
		Total	

Workout	Set	Weight	Reps	Distance	Duration	Calories Burned
					Total	

Daily Workout

Date _____

Goal

Notes

Water ◇◇◇◇◇◇◇◇   Mood 😀 🙂 😊 😐 😓 😵

Meal	Food	Amount	Calories
Breakfast			
Lunch			
Dinner			
Snacks			
		Total	

Workout	Set	Weight	Reps	Distance	Duration	Calories Burned
					Total	

Daily Workout

Date _____

Goal

Notes

Water ◇◇◇◇◇◇◇◇   Mood 😀 🙂 😊 😐 😣 😵

Meal	Food	Amount	Calories
Breakfast			
Lunch			
Dinner			
Snacks			
		Total	

Workout	Set	Weight	Reps	Distance	Duration	Calories Burned
					Total	

Daily Workout

Date _____

Goal

Notes

Water ⬦⬦⬦⬦⬦⬦⬦⬦   Mood 😀 🙂 😊 😐 😣 😵

Meal	Food	Amount	Calories
Breakfast			
Lunch			
Dinner			
Snacks			
		Total	

Workout	Set	Weight	Reps	Distance	Duration	Calories Burned
					Total	

Daily Workout

Date _____

Goal

Notes

Water ⬡⬡⬡⬡⬡⬡⬡⬡

Mood 😃 🙂 😊 😐 😰 😵

Meal	Food	Amount	Calories
Breakfast			
Lunch			
Dinner			
Snacks			
		Total	

Workout	Set	Weight	Reps	Distance	Duration	Calories Burned
					Total	

Daily Workout

Date _____

Goal

Notes

Water ⬦⬦⬦⬦⬦⬦⬦   Mood 😀 🙂 😅 😑 😓 😖

Meal	Food	Amount	Calories
Breakfast			
Lunch			
Dinner			
Snacks			
		Total	

Workout	Set	Weight	Reps	Distance	Duration	Calories Burned
					Total	

Weekly check in

Week of _____

Goals

Notes

	Mon	Tue	Wed	Thu	Fri	Sat	Sun
Cardio	☐	☐	☐	☐	☐	☐	☐
Arms	☐	☐	☐	☐	☐	☐	☐
Abs and Obliques	☐	☐	☐	☐	☐	☐	☐
Lower body	☐	☐	☐	☐	☐	☐	☐
Rest	☐	☐	☐	☐	☐	☐	☐
Water	☐	☐	☐	☐	☐	☐	☐
Healthy food	☐	☐	☐	☐	☐	☐	☐
	☐	☐	☐	☐	☐	☐	☐
	☐	☐	☐	☐	☐	☐	☐
	☐	☐	☐	☐	☐	☐	☐

	Starting	Ending	Difference	Notes
Weight				
Arms				
Chest				
Waist				
Hips				
Thighs				

Daily Workout

Date _____

Goal

Notes

Water ⬡ ⬡ ⬡ ⬡ ⬡ ⬡ ⬡ ⬡   Mood 😀 🙂 😊 😐 😫 😵

Meal	Food	Amount	Calories
Breakfast			
Lunch			
Dinner			
Snacks			
		Total	

Workout	Set	Weight	Reps	Distance	Duration	Calories Burned
					Total	

Daily Workout

Date _____

Goal

Notes

Water 〇〇〇〇〇〇〇〇   Mood 😀 🙂 😊 😑 😖 😵

Meal	Food	Amount	Calories
Breakfast			
Lunch			
Dinner			
Snacks			
		Total	

Workout	Set	Weight	Reps	Distance	Duration	Calories Burned
					Total	

Daily Workout

Date _____

Goal

Notes

Water ◇◇◇◇◇◇◇◇   Mood 😀 🙂 😊 😑 😣 😖

Meal	Food	Amount	Calories
Breakfast			
Lunch			
Dinner			
Snacks			
		Total	

Workout	Set	Weight	Reps	Distance	Duration	Calories Burned
					Total	

Daily Workout

Date _____

Goal

Notes

Water 〇 〇 〇 〇 〇 〇 〇 〇   Mood 😃 🙂 😊 😌 😵 😖

Meal	Food	Amount	Calories
Breakfast			
Lunch			
Dinner			
Snacks			
		Total	

Workout	Set	Weight	Reps	Distance	Duration	Calories Burned
					Total	

Daily Workout

Date _____

Goal

Notes

Water ⬦⬦⬦⬦⬦⬦⬦   Mood 😀 🙂 😊 😑 😣 😨

Meal	Food	Amount	Calories
Breakfast			
Lunch			
Dinner			
Snacks			
		Total	

Workout	Set	Weight	Reps	Distance	Duration	Calories Burned
					Total	

Daily Workout

Date _____

Goal

Notes

Water ⬡ ⬡ ⬡ ⬡ ⬡ ⬡ ⬡   **Mood** 😀 🙂 😊 😒 😰 😵

Meal	Food	Amount	Calories
Breakfast			
Lunch			
Dinner			
Snacks			
		Total	

Workout	Set	Weight	Reps	Distance	Duration	Calories Burned
					Total	

Daily Workout

Date _____

Goal

Notes

Water ⬡⬡⬡⬡⬡⬡⬡

Mood 😃 🙂 😊 😐 😓 😖

Meal	Food	Amount	Calories
Breakfast			
Lunch			
Dinner			
Snacks			
		Total	

Workout	Set	Weight	Reps	Distance	Duration	Calories Burned
					Total	

Weekly check in

Goals	Notes

	Mon	Tue	Wed	Thu	Fri	Sat	Sun
Cardio	☐	☐	☐	☐	☐	☐	☐
Arms	☐	☐	☐	☐	☐	☐	☐
Abs and Obliques	☐	☐	☐	☐	☐	☐	☐
Lower body	☐	☐	☐	☐	☐	☐	☐
Rest	☐	☐	☐	☐	☐	☐	☐
Water	☐	☐	☐	☐	☐	☐	☐
Healthy food	☐	☐	☐	☐	☐	☐	☐
	☐	☐	☐	☐	☐	☐	☐
	☐	☐	☐	☐	☐	☐	☐
	☐	☐	☐	☐	☐	☐	☐

	Starting	Ending	Difference	Notes
Weight				
Arms				
Chest				
Waist				
Hips				
Thighs				

Daily Workout

Date _____

Goal	Notes

Water ◇◇◇◇◇◇◇◇   Mood 😀 🙂 😊 😔 😣 😖

Meal	Food	Amount	Calories
Breakfast			
Lunch			
Dinner			
Snacks			
		Total	

Workout	Set	Weight	Reps	Distance	Duration	Calories Burned
					Total	

Daily Workout

Date _____

Goal

Notes

Water ⬡ ⬡ ⬡ ⬡ ⬡ ⬡ ⬡ ⬡   Mood 😀 🙂 😊 😑 😓 😵

Meal	Food	Amount	Calories
Breakfast			
Lunch			
Dinner			
Snacks			
		Total	

Workout	Set	Weight	Reps	Distance	Duration	Calories Burned
					Total	

Daily Workout

Date _____

Goal

Notes

Water ⬦⬦⬦⬦⬦⬦⬦   Mood 😀 🙂 😊 😣 😰 😵

Meal	Food	Amount	Calories
Breakfast			
Lunch			
Dinner			
Snacks			
		Total	

Workout	Set	Weight	Reps	Distance	Duration	Calories Burned
					Total	

Daily Workout

Date _____

Goal

Notes

Water ◇ ◇ ◇ ◇ ◇ ◇ ◇ ◇   Mood 😀 🙂 😊 😐 😓 😵

Meal	Food	Amount	Calories
Breakfast			
Lunch			
Dinner			
Snacks			
		Total	

Workout	Set	Weight	Reps	Distance	Duration	Calories Burned
					Total	

Daily Workout

Date _____

Goal

Notes

Water ◇ ◇ ◇ ◇ ◇ ◇ ◇ ◇   Mood 😀 🙂 😊 😒 😰 😵

Meal	Food	Amount	Calories
Breakfast			
Lunch			
Dinner			
Snacks			
		Total	

Workout	Set	Weight	Reps	Distance	Duration	Calories Burned
					Total	

Daily Workout

Date _____

Goal	Notes

Water ◊ ◊ ◊ ◊ ◊ ◊ ◊ ◊   Mood 😀 🙂 😊 😑 😰 😵

Meal	Food	Amount	Calories
Breakfast			
Lunch			
Dinner			
Snacks			
		Total	

Workout	Set	Weight	Reps	Distance	Duration	Calories Burned
					Total	

Daily Workout

Date _____

Goal _____

Notes

Water ⬭ ⬭ ⬭ ⬭ ⬭ ⬭ ⬭ ⬭   Mood 😀 🙂 😊 😑 😣 😵

Meal	Food	Amount	Calories
Breakfast			
Lunch			
Dinner			
Snacks			
		Total	

Workout	Set	Weight	Reps	Distance	Duration	Calories Burned
					Total	

Weekly check in

Week of _____

Goals

Notes

	Mon	Tue	Wed	Thu	Fri	Sat	Sun
Cardio	☐	☐	☐	☐	☐	☐	☐
Arms	☐	☐	☐	☐	☐	☐	☐
Abs and Obliques	☐	☐	☐	☐	☐	☐	☐
Lower body	☐	☐	☐	☐	☐	☐	☐
Rest	☐	☐	☐	☐	☐	☐	☐
Water	☐	☐	☐	☐	☐	☐	☐
Healthy food	☐	☐	☐	☐	☐	☐	☐
	☐	☐	☐	☐	☐	☐	☐
	☐	☐	☐	☐	☐	☐	☐
	☐	☐	☐	☐	☐	☐	☐

	Starting	Ending	Difference	Notes
Weight				
Arms				
Chest				
Waist				
Hips				
Thighs				

Daily Workout

Date _____

Goal

Notes

Water ⬡ ⬡ ⬡ ⬡ ⬡ ⬡ ⬡ ⬡   Mood 😀 🙂 😊 😑 😰 😵

Meal	Food	Amount	Calories
Breakfast			
Lunch			
Dinner			
Snacks			
		Total	

Workout	Set	Weight	Reps	Distance	Duration	Calories Burned
					Total	

Daily Workout

Date _____

Goal	Notes

Water ⬡⬡⬡⬡⬡⬡⬡   Mood 😀 🙂 😊 😣 😰 😵

Meal	Food	Amount	Calories
Breakfast			
Lunch			
Dinner			
Snacks			
		Total	

Workout	Set	Weight	Reps	Distance	Duration	Calories Burned
					Total	

Daily Workout

Date _____

Goal

Notes

Water ⬭ ⬭ ⬭ ⬭ ⬭ ⬭ ⬭   Mood 😀 🙂 😅 😕 😣 😖

Meal	Food	Amount	Calories
Breakfast			
Lunch			
Dinner			
Snacks			
		Total	

Workout	Set	Weight	Reps	Distance	Duration	Calories Burned
					Total	

Daily Workout

Date _____

Goal

Notes

Water ◇ ◇ ◇ ◇ ◇ ◇ ◇ ◇   Mood 😀 🙂 😊 😐 😵 😖

Meal	Food	Amount	Calories
Breakfast			
Lunch			
Dinner			
Snacks			
		Total	

Workout	Set	Weight	Reps	Distance	Duration	Calories Burned
					Total	

Daily Workout

Date _____

Goal	Notes

Water ⬦⬦⬦⬦⬦⬦⬦⬦   Mood 😀 🙂 😊 😐 😣 😖

Meal	Food	Amount	Calories
Breakfast			
Lunch			
Dinner			
Snacks			
		Total	

Workout	Set	Weight	Reps	Distance	Duration	Calories Burned
					Total	

Daily Workout

Date _____

Goal	Notes

Water ◊ ◊ ◊ ◊ ◊ ◊ ◊ ◊   Mood 😀 🙂 😊 😌 😰 😵

Meal	Food	Amount	Calories
Breakfast			
Lunch			
Dinner			
Snacks			
		Total	

Workout	Set	Weight	Reps	Distance	Duration	Calories Burned
					Total	

Daily Workout

Date _____

Goal

Notes

Water ⬦ ⬦ ⬦ ⬦ ⬦ ⬦ ⬦   Mood 😃 🙂 😌 😔 😣 😖

Meal	Food	Amount	Calories
Breakfast			
Lunch			
Dinner			
Snacks			
		Total	

Workout	Set	Weight	Reps	Distance	Duration	Calories Burned
					Total	

Weekly check in

Week of _____

Goals

Notes

	Mon	Tue	Wed	Thu	Fri	Sat	Sun
Cardio	☐	☐	☐	☐	☐	☐	☐
Arms	☐	☐	☐	☐	☐	☐	☐
Abs and Obliques	☐	☐	☐	☐	☐	☐	☐
Lower body	☐	☐	☐	☐	☐	☐	☐
Rest	☐	☐	☐	☐	☐	☐	☐
Water	☐	☐	☐	☐	☐	☐	☐
Healthy food	☐	☐	☐	☐	☐	☐	☐
	☐	☐	☐	☐	☐	☐	☐
	☐	☐	☐	☐	☐	☐	☐
	☐	☐	☐	☐	☐	☐	☐

	Starting	Ending	Difference	Notes
Weight				
Arms				
Chest				
Waist				
Hips				
Thighs				

Daily Workout

Date _____

Goal

Notes

Water ⬡ ⬡ ⬡ ⬡ ⬡ ⬡ ⬡   Mood 😃 🙂 😊 😐 😓 😖

Meal	Food	Amount	Calories
Breakfast			
Lunch			
Dinner			
Snacks			
		Total	

Workout	Set	Weight	Reps	Distance	Duration	Calories Burned
					Total	

Daily Workout

Date _____

Goal

Notes

Water ◇◇◇◇◇◇◇◇   Mood 😃 🙂 😊 😓 😰 😵

Meal	Food	Amount	Calories
Breakfast			
Lunch			
Dinner			
Snacks			
		Total	

Workout	Set	Weight	Reps	Distance	Duration	Calories Burned
					Total	

Daily Workout

Date _____

Goal

Notes

Water ⬡ ⬡ ⬡ ⬡ ⬡ ⬡ ⬡ ⬡   Mood 😀 🙂 😊 😑 😫 😵

Meal	Food	Amount	Calories
Breakfast			
Lunch			
Dinner			
Snacks			
		Total	

Workout	Set	Weight	Reps	Distance	Duration	Calories Burned
					Total	

Daily Workout

Date _____

Goal

Notes

Water ⬦⬦⬦⬦⬦⬦⬦⬦ Mood 😀 🙂 😊 😑 😓 😵

Meal	Food	Amount	Calories
Breakfast			
Lunch			
Dinner			
Snacks			
		Total	

Workout	Set	Weight	Reps	Distance	Duration	Calories Burned
					Total	

Daily Workout

Date _____

Goal

Notes

Water ⬦⬦⬦⬦⬦⬦⬦⬦   Mood 😀 🙂 😊 😣 😰 😫

Meal	Food	Amount	Calories
Breakfast			
Lunch			
Dinner			
Snacks			
		Total	

Workout	Set	Weight	Reps	Distance	Duration	Calories Burned
					Total	

Daily Workout

Date _____

Goal

Notes

Water ◇ ◇ ◇ ◇ ◇ ◇ ◇ ◇   Mood 🙂 🙂 😊 😑 😓 😵

Meal	Food	Amount	Calories
Breakfast			
Lunch			
Dinner			
Snacks			
		Total	

Workout	Set	Weight	Reps	Distance	Duration	Calories Burned
					Total	

Daily Workout

Date _____

Goal

Notes

Water ◇ ◇ ◇ ◇ ◇ ◇ ◇ ◇   Mood 😀 🙂 😊 😑 😓 😖

Meal	Food	Amount	Calories
Breakfast			
Lunch			
Dinner			
Snacks			
		Total	

Workout	Set	Weight	Reps	Distance	Duration	Calories Burned
					Total	

Weekly check in

Week of _____

Goals	Notes

	Mon	Tue	Wed	Thu	Fri	Sat	Sun
Cardio	☐	☐	☐	☐	☐	☐	☐
Arms	☐	☐	☐	☐	☐	☐	☐
Abs and Obliques	☐	☐	☐	☐	☐	☐	☐
Lower body	☐	☐	☐	☐	☐	☐	☐
Rest	☐	☐	☐	☐	☐	☐	☐
Water	☐	☐	☐	☐	☐	☐	☐
Healthy food	☐	☐	☐	☐	☐	☐	☐
	☐	☐	☐	☐	☐	☐	☐
	☐	☐	☐	☐	☐	☐	☐
	☐	☐	☐	☐	☐	☐	☐

	Starting	Ending	Difference	Notes
Weight				
Arms				
Chest				
Waist				
Hips				
Thighs				

Daily Workout

Date _____

Goal	Notes

Water ◇◇◇◇◇◇◇◇   Mood 😀 🙂 😊 😑 😖 😵

Meal	Food	Amount	Calories
Breakfast			
Lunch			
Dinner			
Snacks			
		Total	

Workout	Set	Weight	Reps	Distance	Duration	Calories Burned
					Total	

Daily Workout

Date _____

Goal

Notes

Water 〇〇〇〇〇〇〇〇   Mood 😀 🙂 😊 😑 😰 😵

Meal	Food	Amount	Calories
Breakfast			
Lunch			
Dinner			
Snacks			
		Total	

Workout	Set	Weight	Reps	Distance	Duration	Calories Burned
					Total	

Daily Workout

Date _____

Goal	Notes

Water ⬡ ⬡ ⬡ ⬡ ⬡ ⬡ ⬡ ⬡   Mood 😃 🙂 😊 😑 😣 😵

Meal	Food	Amount	Calories
Breakfast			
Lunch			
Dinner			
Snacks			
		Total	

Workout	Set	Weight	Reps	Distance	Duration	Calories Burned
					Total	

Daily Workout

Date _____

Goal

Notes

Water ◇ ◇ ◇ ◇ ◇ ◇ ◇ ◇   Mood 😀 🙂 😊 😣 😓 😵

Meal	Food	Amount	Calories
Breakfast			
Lunch			
Dinner			
Snacks			
		Total	

Workout	Set	Weight	Reps	Distance	Duration	Calories Burned
					Total	

Daily Workout

Date _____

Goal	Notes

Water ◇◇◇◇◇◇◇◇   Mood 😀 🙂 😌 😒 😣 😵

Meal	Food	Amount	Calories
Breakfast			
Lunch			
Dinner			
Snacks			
		Total	

Workout	Set	Weight	Reps	Distance	Duration	Calories Burned
					Total	

Daily Workout

Date _____

Goal

Notes

Water ⬡ ⬡ ⬡ ⬡ ⬡ ⬡ ⬡ ⬡   Mood 😀 🙂 😊 😑 😵 😖

Meal	Food	Amount	Calories
Breakfast			
Lunch			
Dinner			
Snacks			
		Total	

Workout	Set	Weight	Reps	Distance	Duration	Calories Burned
					Total	

Daily Workout

Date _____

Goal

Notes

Water ⬡ ⬡ ⬡ ⬡ ⬡ ⬡ ⬡ Mood 😀 🙂 😊 😑 😖 😵

Meal	Food	Amount	Calories
Breakfast			
Lunch			
Dinner			
Snacks			
		Total	

Workout	Set	Weight	Reps	Distance	Duration	Calories Burned
					Total	

Weekly check in

Week of _____

Goals

Notes

	Mon	Tue	Wed	Thu	Fri	Sat	Sun
Cardio	☐	☐	☐	☐	☐	☐	☐
Arms	☐	☐	☐	☐	☐	☐	☐
Abs and Obliques	☐	☐	☐	☐	☐	☐	☐
Lower body	☐	☐	☐	☐	☐	☐	☐
Rest	☐	☐	☐	☐	☐	☐	☐
Water	☐	☐	☐	☐	☐	☐	☐
Healthy food	☐	☐	☐	☐	☐	☐	☐
	☐	☐	☐	☐	☐	☐	☐
	☐	☐	☐	☐	☐	☐	☐
	☐	☐	☐	☐	☐	☐	☐

	Starting	Ending	Difference	Notes
Weight				
Arms				
Chest				
Waist				
Hips				
Thighs				

Daily Workout

Date _____

Goal

Notes

Water ⬭⬭⬭⬭⬭⬭⬭⬭   Mood 😃 🙂 😊 😒 😰 😖

Meal	Food	Amount	Calories
Breakfast			
Lunch			
Dinner			
Snacks			
		Total	

Workout	Set	Weight	Reps	Distance	Duration	Calories Burned
					Total	

Daily Workout

Date _____

Goal

Notes

Water ◊ ◊ ◊ ◊ ◊ ◊ ◊ ◊   Mood   😀   🙂   😊   😔   😰   😵

Meal	Food	Amount	Calories
Breakfast			
Lunch			
Dinner			
Snacks			
		Total	

Workout	Set	Weight	Reps	Distance	Duration	Calories Burned
					Total	

Daily Workout

Date _____

Goal

Notes

Water ◇◇◇◇◇◇◇◇   Mood 😀 🙂 😊 😒 😣 😖

Meal	Food	Amount	Calories
Breakfast			
Lunch			
Dinner			
Snacks			
		Total	

Workout	Set	Weight	Reps	Distance	Duration	Calories Burned
					Total	

Daily Workout

Date _____

Goal

Notes

Water ◇ ◇ ◇ ◇ ◇ ◇ ◇ ◇   Mood 😀 🙂 😊 😑 😣 😵

Meal	Food	Amount	Calories
Breakfast			
Lunch			
Dinner			
Snacks			
		Total	

Workout	Set	Weight	Reps	Distance	Duration	Calories Burned
					Total	

Daily Workout

Date _____

Goal

Notes

Water ◊◊◊◊◊◊◊◊   Mood 😀 🙂 😊 😑 😣 😷

Meal	Food	Amount	Calories
Breakfast			
Lunch			
Dinner			
Snacks			
		Total	

Workout	Set	Weight	Reps	Distance	Duration	Calories Burned
					Total	

Daily Workout

Date _____

Goal

Notes

Water ◇◇◇◇◇◇◇◇   Mood 😃 🙂 😊 😒 😣 😵

Meal	Food	Amount	Calories
Breakfast			
Lunch			
Dinner			
Snacks			
		Total	

Workout	Set	Weight	Reps	Distance	Duration	Calories Burned
					Total	

Daily Workout

Date _____

Goal	Notes

Water ⬦⬦⬦⬦⬦⬦⬦⬦   Mood 😀 🙂 😊 😑 😖 😵

Meal	Food	Amount	Calories
Breakfast			
Lunch			
Dinner			
Snacks			
		Total	

Workout	Set	Weight	Reps	Distance	Duration	Calories Burned
					Total	

Weekly check in

Week of _____

Goals

Notes

	Mon	Tue	Wed	Thu	Fri	Sat	Sun
Cardio	☐	☐	☐	☐	☐	☐	☐
Arms	☐	☐	☐	☐	☐	☐	☐
Abs and Obliques	☐	☐	☐	☐	☐	☐	☐
Lower body	☐	☐	☐	☐	☐	☐	☐
Rest	☐	☐	☐	☐	☐	☐	☐
Water	☐	☐	☐	☐	☐	☐	☐
Healthy food	☐	☐	☐	☐	☐	☐	☐
	☐	☐	☐	☐	☐	☐	☐
	☐	☐	☐	☐	☐	☐	☐
	☐	☐	☐	☐	☐	☐	☐

	Starting	Ending	Difference	Notes
Weight				
Arms				
Chest				
Waist				
Hips				
Thighs				

Daily Workout

Date _____

Goal

Notes

Water ⬭⬭⬭⬭⬭⬭⬭⬭   Mood 😀 🙂 😊 😐 😓 😖

Meal	Food	Amount	Calories
Breakfast			
Lunch			
Dinner			
Snacks			
		Total	

Workout	Set	Weight	Reps	Distance	Duration	Calories Burned
					Total	

Daily Workout

Date _____

Goal	Notes

Water ◇ ◇ ◇ ◇ ◇ ◇ ◇ ◇   Mood 😀 🙂 😊 😑 😵 😖

Meal	Food	Amount	Calories
Breakfast			
Lunch			
Dinner			
Snacks			
		Total	

Workout	Set	Weight	Reps	Distance	Duration	Calories Burned
					Total	

Daily Workout

Date _____

Goal

Notes

Water ⬡⬡⬡⬡⬡⬡⬡⬡   Mood 😀 🙂 😊 😑 😖 😵

Meal	Food	Amount	Calories
Breakfast			
Lunch			
Dinner			
Snacks			
		Total	

Workout	Set	Weight	Reps	Distance	Duration	Calories Burned
					Total	

Daily Workout

Date _____

Goal

Notes

Water ⬡ ⬡ ⬡ ⬡ ⬡ ⬡ ⬡ ⬡   Mood 😀 🙂 😊 😐 😣 😵

Meal	Food	Amount	Calories
Breakfast			
Lunch			
Dinner			
Snacks			
		Total	

Workout	Set	Weight	Reps	Distance	Duration	Calories Burned
					Total	

Daily Workout

Date _____

Goal

Notes

Water ⬡ ⬡ ⬡ ⬡ ⬡ ⬡ ⬡ ⬡   Mood 😀 🙂 😊 😑 😰 😵

Meal	Food	Amount	Calories
Breakfast			
Lunch			
Dinner			
Snacks			
		Total	

Workout	Set	Weight	Reps	Distance	Duration	Calories Burned
					Total	

Daily Workout

Date _____

Goal

Notes

Water ◊ ◊ ◊ ◊ ◊ ◊ ◊ ◊   Mood 😃 🙂 😊 😓 😖 😵

Meal	Food	Amount	Calories
Breakfast			
Lunch			
Dinner			
Snacks			
		Total	

Workout	Set	Weight	Reps	Distance	Duration	Calories Burned
					Total	

Daily Workout

Date _____

Goal

Notes

Water ⬨⬨⬨⬨⬨⬨⬨   Mood 😀 🙂 😊 😐 😓 😖

Meal	Food	Amount	Calories
Breakfast			
Lunch			
Dinner			
Snacks			
		Total	

Workout	Set	Weight	Reps	Distance	Duration	Calories Burned
					Total	

Weekly check in

Week of _____

Goals

Notes

	Mon	Tue	Wed	Thu	Fri	Sat	Sun
Cardio	☐	☐	☐	☐	☐	☐	☐
Arms	☐	☐	☐	☐	☐	☐	☐
Abs and Obliques	☐	☐	☐	☐	☐	☐	☐
Lower body	☐	☐	☐	☐	☐	☐	☐
Rest	☐	☐	☐	☐	☐	☐	☐
Water	☐	☐	☐	☐	☐	☐	☐
Healthy food	☐	☐	☐	☐	☐	☐	☐
	☐	☐	☐	☐	☐	☐	☐
	☐	☐	☐	☐	☐	☐	☐
	☐	☐	☐	☐	☐	☐	☐

	Starting	Ending	Difference	Notes
Weight				
Arms				
Chest				
Waist				
Hips				
Thighs				

Daily Workout

Date _____

Goal

Notes

Water ⬦ ⬦ ⬦ ⬦ ⬦ ⬦ ⬦ ⬦   Mood 😃 🙂 😅 😓 😵 😖

Meal	Food	Amount	Calories
Breakfast			
Lunch			
Dinner			
Snacks			
		Total	

Workout	Set	Weight	Reps	Distance	Duration	Calories Burned
					Total	

Daily Workout

Date _____

Goal

Notes

Water ◇◇◇◇◇◇◇◇   Mood 😀 🙂 😊 😐 😫 😵

Meal	Food	Amount	Calories
Breakfast			
Lunch			
Dinner			
Snacks			
		Total	

Workout	Set	Weight	Reps	Distance	Duration	Calories Burned
					Total	

Daily Workout

Date _____

Goal	Notes

Water ◇ ◇ ◇ ◇ ◇ ◇ ◇ ◇   Mood 😀 🙂 😊 😑 😖 😵

Meal	Food	Amount	Calories
Breakfast			
Lunch			
Dinner			
Snacks			
		Total	

Workout	Set	Weight	Reps	Distance	Duration	Calories Burned
					Total	

Daily Workout

Date _____

Goal

Notes

Water 〇〇〇〇〇〇〇〇   Mood 😀 🙂 😅 😑 😰 😵

Meal	Food	Amount	Calories
Breakfast			
Lunch			
Dinner			
Snacks			
		Total	

Workout	Set	Weight	Reps	Distance	Duration	Calories Burned
					Total	

Daily Workout

Date _____

Goal

Notes

Water ⬡⬡⬡⬡⬡⬡⬡⬡   Mood 😀 🙂 😊 😐 😫 😖

Meal	Food	Amount	Calories
Breakfast			
Lunch			
Dinner			
Snacks			
		Total	

Workout	Set	Weight	Reps	Distance	Duration	Calories Burned
					Total	

Daily Workout

Date _____

Goal

Notes

Water ◇◇◇◇◇◇◇◇   Mood 😃 🙂 😅 😒 😓 😖

Meal	Food	Amount	Calories
Breakfast			
Lunch			
Dinner			
Snacks			
		Total	

Workout	Set	Weight	Reps	Distance	Duration	Calories Burned
					Total	

Daily Workout

Date _____

Goal

Notes

Water ⬡ ⬡ ⬡ ⬡ ⬡ ⬡ ⬡   Mood 😀 🙂 😊 😓 😣 😵

Meal	Food	Amount	Calories
Breakfast			
Lunch			
Dinner			
Snacks			
		Total	

Workout	Set	Weight	Reps	Distance	Duration	Calories Burned
					Total	

Weekly check in

Week of _____

Goals

Notes

	Mon	Tue	Wed	Thu	Fri	Sat	Sun
Cardio	☐	☐	☐	☐	☐	☐	☐
Arms	☐	☐	☐	☐	☐	☐	☐
Abs and Obliques	☐	☐	☐	☐	☐	☐	☐
Lower body	☐	☐	☐	☐	☐	☐	☐
Rest	☐	☐	☐	☐	☐	☐	☐
Water	☐	☐	☐	☐	☐	☐	☐
Healthy food	☐	☐	☐	☐	☐	☐	☐
	☐	☐	☐	☐	☐	☐	☐
	☐	☐	☐	☐	☐	☐	☐
	☐	☐	☐	☐	☐	☐	☐

	Starting	Ending	Difference	Notes
Weight				
Arms				
Chest				
Waist				
Hips				
Thighs				

Daily Workout

Date _____

Goal

Notes

Water ⬙⬙⬙⬙⬙⬙⬙⬙   Mood 😃 🙂 😊 😑 😰 😵

Meal	Food	Amount	Calories
Breakfast			
Lunch			
Dinner			
Snacks			
		Total	

Workout	Set	Weight	Reps	Distance	Duration	Calories Burned
					Total	

Daily Workout

Date _____

Goal

Notes

Water ⬦⬦⬦⬦⬦⬦⬦⬦ Mood 😀 🙂 😊 😑 😓 😖

Meal	Food	Amount	Calories
Breakfast			
Lunch			
Dinner			
Snacks			
		Total	

Workout	Set	Weight	Reps	Distance	Duration	Calories Burned
					Total	

Daily Workout

Date _____

Goal

Notes

Water ⬡⬡⬡⬡⬡⬡⬡ Mood 😀 🙂 😅 😑 😣 😰

Meal	Food	Amount	Calories
Breakfast			
Lunch			
Dinner			
Snacks			
		Total	

Workout	Set	Weight	Reps	Distance	Duration	Calories Burned
					Total	

Daily Workout

Date _____

Goal

Notes

Water ⬡⬡⬡⬡⬡⬡⬡⬡   Mood 😀 🙂 😊 😑 😓 😵

Meal	Food	Amount	Calories
Breakfast			
Lunch			
Dinner			
Snacks			
		Total	

Workout	Set	Weight	Reps	Distance	Duration	Calories Burned
					Total	

Daily Workout

Date _____

Goal	Notes

Water ◇ ◇ ◇ ◇ ◇ ◇ ◇ ◇   Mood 😀 🙂 😌 😓 😖 😵

Meal	Food	Amount	Calories
Breakfast			
Lunch			
Dinner			
Snacks			
		Total	

Workout	Set	Weight	Reps	Distance	Duration	Calories Burned
					Total	

Daily Workout

Date _____

Goal

Notes

Water ⬦ ⬦ ⬦ ⬦ ⬦ ⬦ ⬦ ⬦   Mood 😀 🙂 😊 😑 😖 😵

Meal	Food	Amount	Calories
Breakfast			
Lunch			
Dinner			
Snacks			
		Total	

Workout	Set	Weight	Reps	Distance	Duration	Calories Burned
					Total	

Daily Workout

Date _____

Goal

Notes

Water 〇〇〇〇〇〇〇〇   Mood 😃 🙂 😊 😑 😣 😖

Meal	Food	Amount	Calories
Breakfast			
Lunch			
Dinner			
Snacks			
		Total	

Workout	Set	Weight	Reps	Distance	Duration	Calories Burned
					Total	

Weekly check in

Week of _____

Goals

Notes

	Mon	Tue	Wed	Thu	Fri	Sat	Sun
Cardio	☐	☐	☐	☐	☐	☐	☐
Arms	☐	☐	☐	☐	☐	☐	☐
Abs and Obliques	☐	☐	☐	☐	☐	☐	☐
Lower body	☐	☐	☐	☐	☐	☐	☐
Rest	☐	☐	☐	☐	☐	☐	☐
Water	☐	☐	☐	☐	☐	☐	☐
Healthy food	☐	☐	☐	☐	☐	☐	☐
	☐	☐	☐	☐	☐	☐	☐
	☐	☐	☐	☐	☐	☐	☐
	☐	☐	☐	☐	☐	☐	☐

	Starting	Ending	Difference	Notes
Weight				
Arms				
Chest				
Waist				
Hips				
Thighs				

Daily Workout

Date _____

Goal	Notes

Water ◇ ◇ ◇ ◇ ◇ ◇ ◇ ◇   Mood 😀 🙂 😊 😐 😫 😵

Meal	Food	Amount	Calories
Breakfast			
Lunch			
Dinner			
Snacks			
		Total	

Workout	Set	Weight	Reps	Distance	Duration	Calories Burned
					Total	

Daily Workout

Date _____

Goal

Notes

Water ⬦⬦⬦⬦⬦⬦⬦   Mood 😀 🙂 😅 😓 😵 😖

Meal	Food	Amount	Calories
Breakfast			
Lunch			
Dinner			
Snacks			
		Total	

Workout	Set	Weight	Reps	Distance	Duration	Calories Burned
					Total	

Daily Workout

Date _____

Goal

Notes

Water ⬡⬡⬡⬡⬡⬡⬡⬡   Mood 😀 🙂 😊 😓 😵 😖

Meal	Food	Amount	Calories
Breakfast			
Lunch			
Dinner			
Snacks			
		Total	

Workout	Set	Weight	Reps	Distance	Duration	Calories Burned
					Total	

Daily Workout

Date _____

Goal	Notes

Water ⬡ ⬡ ⬡ ⬡ ⬡ ⬡ ⬡ ⬡   Mood 😀 🙂 😊 😐 😖 😵

Meal	Food	Amount	Calories
Breakfast			
Lunch			
Dinner			
Snacks			
		Total	

Workout	Set	Weight	Reps	Distance	Duration	Calories Burned
					Total	

Daily Workout

Date _____

Goal

Notes

Water ⬦⬦⬦⬦⬦⬦⬦⬦   Mood 😃 🙂 😊 😐 😣 😵

Meal	Food	Amount	Calories
Breakfast			
Lunch			
Dinner			
Snacks			
		Total	

Workout	Set	Weight	Reps	Distance	Duration	Calories Burned
					Total	

Daily Workout

Date _____

Goal

Notes

Water ◊ ◊ ◊ ◊ ◊ ◊ ◊   Mood 😀 🙂 😊 😑 😖 😵

Meal	Food	Amount	Calories
Breakfast			
Lunch			
Dinner			
Snacks			
		Total	

Workout	Set	Weight	Reps	Distance	Duration	Calories Burned
					Total	

Daily Workout

Date _____

Goal

Notes

Water ⬭⬭⬭⬭⬭⬭⬭⬭   Mood 😀 🙂 😄 😑 😫 😵

Meal	Food	Amount	Calories
Breakfast			
Lunch			
Dinner			
Snacks			
		Total	

Workout	Set	Weight	Reps	Distance	Duration	Calories Burned
					Total	

Weekly check in

Week of _____

Goals

Notes

	Mon	Tue	Wed	Thu	Fri	Sat	Sun
Cardio	☐	☐	☐	☐	☐	☐	☐
Arms	☐	☐	☐	☐	☐	☐	☐
Abs and Obliques	☐	☐	☐	☐	☐	☐	☐
Lower body	☐	☐	☐	☐	☐	☐	☐
Rest	☐	☐	☐	☐	☐	☐	☐
Water	☐	☐	☐	☐	☐	☐	☐
Healthy food	☐	☐	☐	☐	☐	☐	☐
	☐	☐	☐	☐	☐	☐	☐
	☐	☐	☐	☐	☐	☐	☐
	☐	☐	☐	☐	☐	☐	☐

	Starting	Ending	Difference	Notes
Weight				
Arms				
Chest				
Waist				
Hips				
Thighs				

Daily Workout

Date _____

Goal

Notes

Water ◇◇◇◇◇◇◇◇   Mood 😀 🙂 😊 😑 😓 😖

Meal	Food	Amount	Calories
Breakfast			
Lunch			
Dinner			
Snacks			
		Total	

Workout	Set	Weight	Reps	Distance	Duration	Calories Burned
					Total	

Daily Workout

Date _____

Goal

Notes

Water ◇ ◇ ◇ ◇ ◇ ◇ ◇ ◇   Mood 😀 🙂 😊 😐 😫 😵

Meal	Food	Amount	Calories
Breakfast			
Lunch			
Dinner			
Snacks			
		Total	

Workout	Set	Weight	Reps	Distance	Duration	Calories Burned
					Total	

Daily Workout

Date _____

Goal	Notes

Water ⬡⬡⬡⬡⬡⬡⬡⬡   Mood 😀 🙂 😊 😑 😫 😵

Meal	Food	Amount	Calories
Breakfast			
Lunch			
Dinner			
Snacks			
		Total	

Workout	Set	Weight	Reps	Distance	Duration	Calories Burned
					Total	

Daily Workout

Date _____

Goal

Notes

Water 〇〇〇〇〇〇〇〇   Mood 😀 🙂 😊 😐 😵 😖

Meal	Food	Amount	Calories
Breakfast			
Lunch			
Dinner			
Snacks			
		Total	

Workout	Set	Weight	Reps	Distance	Duration	Calories Burned
					Total	

Daily Workout

Date _____

Goal

Notes

Water ⬦⬦⬦⬦⬦⬦⬦ Mood 😀 🙂 😊 😔 😫 😵

Meal	Food	Amount	Calories
Breakfast			
Lunch			
Dinner			
Snacks			
		Total	

Workout	Set	Weight	Reps	Distance	Duration	Calories Burned
					Total	

Daily Workout

Date _____

Goal	Notes

Water ◊◊◊◊◊◊◊◊   Mood 😀 🙂 😊 😐 😓 😵

Meal	Food	Amount	Calories
Breakfast			
Lunch			
Dinner			
Snacks			
		Total	

Workout	Set	Weight	Reps	Distance	Duration	Calories Burned
					Total	

Daily Workout

Date _____

Goal

Notes

Water ⬡⬡⬡⬡⬡⬡⬡⬡ Mood 😀 🙂 😊 😑 😖 😵

Meal	Food	Amount	Calories
Breakfast			
Lunch			
Dinner			
Snacks			
		Total	

Workout	Set	Weight	Reps	Distance	Duration	Calories Burned
					Total	

Weekly check in

Week of _____

Goals

Notes

	Mon	Tue	Wed	Thu	Fri	Sat	Sun
Cardio	☐	☐	☐	☐	☐	☐	☐
Arms	☐	☐	☐	☐	☐	☐	☐
Abs and Obliques	☐	☐	☐	☐	☐	☐	☐
Lower body	☐	☐	☐	☐	☐	☐	☐
Rest	☐	☐	☐	☐	☐	☐	☐
Water	☐	☐	☐	☐	☐	☐	☐
Healthy food	☐	☐	☐	☐	☐	☐	☐
	☐	☐	☐	☐	☐	☐	☐
	☐	☐	☐	☐	☐	☐	☐
	☐	☐	☐	☐	☐	☐	☐

	Starting	Ending	Difference	Notes
Weight				
Arms				
Chest				
Waist				
Hips				
Thighs				

Want free goodies?

Thank You!

so much for trying our Workout Planner!
We'd love to hear from you!

If you've found this to be a good book please,
support us and leave a review.

If you have any suggestions or issues with this book, or if
you want to test some of our latest notebooks
please email us.

Send email to:

pickme.readme@gmail.com